How to Make Your Penis BIGGER

The Ultimate Guide to Effectively Enhancing Your Penis

Randy Tutt

Copyright Act of 1976, the scanning, uploading and electronic sharing of any part of this book without the explicit written consent or permission of the publisher constitutes unlawful piracy and the theft of intellectual property.

If you would like to use material or content from this book (other than for review purposes), prior written permission must be obtained from the publisher.

You can contact the publishing company at admin@speedypublishing.com. Thank you for not infringing on the author's rights.

Speedy Publishing LLC (c) 2014
40 E. Main St., #1156
Newark, DE 19711
www.speedypublishing.co

Ordering Information:
Quantity sales; Special discounts are available on quantity purchases by corporations, associations, and others. For details, contact the "Special Sales Department" at the address above.

This is a reprint book.

Manufactured in the United States of America

Table of Contents

Publisher's Notes i

Chapter 1: Does Size Matter? 1

Chapter 2: Male Anatomy Explained 6

Chapter 3: Average or Bigger – Which is Really Better? 11

Chapter 4: Does Size Matter to Women? 15

Chapter 5: A Big Penis Doesn't Automatically Mean Great Sex - Bedroom Tips for All Sizes 18

Chapter 6: Is It Really Possible to Make Your Penis Bigger? 25

Chapter 7: Is Penis Enlargement Surgery an Option? 27

Chapter 8: The Penis Exercise Program 29

Chapter 9: Create an Exercise Schedule for Your Penis 47

Chapter 10: Exercise Can Increase Size and Correct Other Issues 54

Chapter 11: Do Pills, Supplements, and Gadgets Work? 58

Chapter 12: When to Seek Medical Advice 68

Chapter 13: Diet, Exercise and Your Health 73

Chapter 14: Conclusion 82

Publisher's Notes

Disclaimer

This publication is intended to provide helpful and informative material. It is not intended to diagnose, treat, cure, or prevent any health problem or condition, nor is intended to replace the advice of a physician. No action should be taken solely on the contents of this book. Always consult your physician or qualified health-care professional on any matters regarding your health and before adopting any suggestions in this book or drawing inferences from it.

The author and publisher specifically disclaim all responsibility for any liability, loss or risk, personal or otherwise, which is incurred as a consequence, directly or indirectly, from the use or application of any contents of this book.

Any and all product names referenced within this book are the trademarks of their respective owners. None of these owners have sponsored, authorized, endorsed, or approved this book.

Always read all information provided by the manufacturers' product labels before using their products. The author and publisher are not responsible for claims made by manufacturers.

CHAPTER 1: DOES SIZE MATTER?

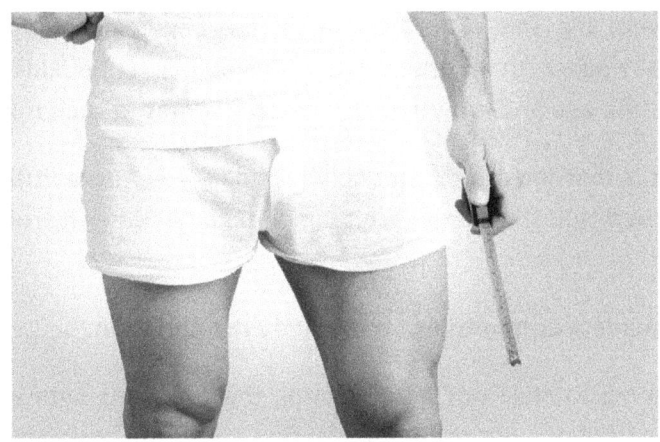

A big penis. If you don't have one, you're not going to do as well in the sex department as guys who have a large member. Is that really true? Do you believe that?

One of the main ways that a man defines himself is by his sex organ. Its size, shape, whether it's straight or it curves left or right, up or down. Logically, this might seem pretty prehistoric, but it's the way it is. Because the biological function of a man is to reproduce, it's necessary to have a sexual organ that will help make you more attractive to the opposite sex.

Yes, in these modern days, spreading your seed around everywhere is frowned upon, but you are still biologically hard-wired to look to your penis as the instrument that you would do that with, and that makes you, and every man, very sensitive about the size of your penis, and how well it functions.

Besides that, your penis and your testicles are the most obvious signs of your manhood, your manliness, your masculinity, and your physical ability to please a woman when it comes to sex.

Chances are, you've always been fascinated by your penis – since you were a little boy. That's normal. And if you happened to see your dad's or big brother's as a tot, you probably wondered why theirs were big and yours was small (the beginning of the "my organ is smaller than other men's" complex). Little kids don't consider the age and growth factor when it comes to such things.

The fact is that most men, possibly including you, are a little (or a lot) worried that their organ isn't big enough, whether it truly is or isn't.

You've made a Commitment to Remedy the Situation

We're going to start out by discussing the problems with a small penis, and follow with some information about the male anatomy. Yes, you already know about the male anatomy – you have all the parts and are quite familiar with them. Trust me; the information will come in handy later.

Although this is a book about how to make your penis grow larger and enhance your sexual experience and prowess all the way around, we do need to talk about whether or not bigger is really better.

You need to consider what bigger is, and how it will make a difference in your life. You also need to consider whether or not you're actually okay the way you are, because it's just possible that there is nothing at all wrong with your size.

Moving on, we'll look at the female perspective – after all, one of your biggest motivations for buying and reading this book is to be more sexually pleasing to your partner, isn't it? If she's happy, you're going to be happy.

We'll also talk about whether or not you really can make it bigger. The answer is yes, by the way, but you have to understand a few things about the process and what realistic expectations should be.

For example, you're not going to turn into King Kong! However, you can increase size when you follow the exercise program, which is the section of the book that outlines the exact exercises you need to do, with complete instructions.

I want to point out here that there is a time factor involved in increasing both girth and length. Sadly, you're not going to do some exercises one day, maybe take a supplement, and then wake the next morning to find that your member has increased noticeably. The growth changes happen gradually, and over a period of weeks and months.

Finally, we'll go over some other ideas for increasing size and stamina including supplements and over the counter medications, and gadgets, the issue of not being able to "get it up," and premature ejaculation.

The point is to help you fully understand the small penis issue and deal with it head on (excuse the pun). If you're having confidence issues in other areas, we're going to address and solve those, too.

The result will be a sexier, stronger, and more confident you - enjoying a sex organ that you feel great about!

The Problem with a Small Penis (What's the Big Deal?)

The problem with a small penis is confidence. The only thing a small penis can and will do to you is ruin your self-esteem and make you feel nervous in the bedroom.

A small penis won't keep you from having children if you want them. It won't keep you from doing your job, fixing your car, paying your bills, or enjoying a tailgate party. And it won't ruin your golf swing.

But if you feel that your penis is small, it will ruin your self-confidence when it comes to changing in the locker room, or getting naked in front of a woman. And those things are a big deal!

If you lack self-confidence when it comes to your sexual organ, you're probably already spending plenty of time and energy avoiding situations where someone, male or female, will see your little guy and possibly make fun of him.

There's not much worse than having someone make a snide comment about the size of your penis, or laugh at it. That's your manhood right there, and this is not a laughing matter!

So if you're avoiding working out at the gym because you don't want the other guys to see your smallish organ, you're doing yourself a huge disservice. You're inhibiting your health and fitness all because of fear and shame.

And if you're not asking women out on dates, or you're shying away from having sex with your partner because she's made some sort of comment about your penis, or she doesn't seem satisfied, you're doing yourself another huge disservice.

Part of the joy of life is sex. If you don't date, or find a partner to have sex with, you're either going to be very frustrated and unhappy, or your arm and hand muscles are going to be very, very strong (and not because you've been to the gym).

Another confidence issue that crops up as a result of having a smaller than usual penis is that you subconsciously might let that issue seep into other areas of your life, such as business and recreation. If you feel like you're not manly enough in the penis area, you might subconsciously feel like you're not capable of handling any situation that requires manly confidence.

Just so you know, there is nothing technically wrong with having a small penis, so long as it performs the functions it was made to do, which are to pass urine out of your body and eject semen for the sake of reproducing the human race.

The problem occurs when you're embarrassed by its tiny size, and afraid that someone is going to find out just how little it is and judge you for it.

Here's a myth about penis size: Penis size is dictated by body size, or the size of hands or feet. That's a myth, so never make assumptions about someone's penis size based on height or frame.

CHAPTER 2: MALE ANATOMY EXPLAINED

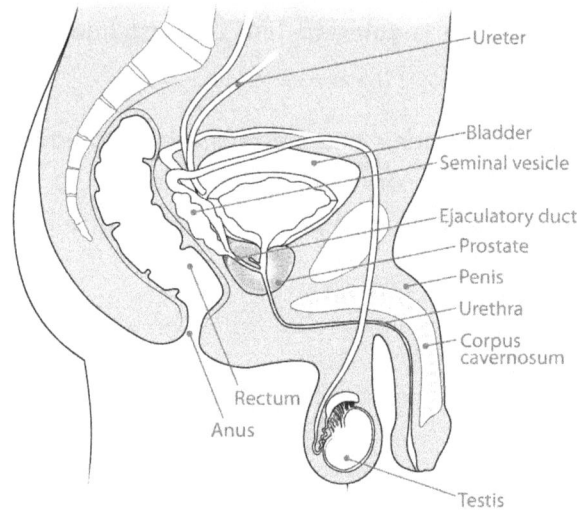

Why do I have to read about my own anatomy?" I'll tell you why. It's because the more you understand how you're put together and how all that stuff works, the better you'll be at getting it to look and work the way you want it to.

Your sex organs and all the underlying tissues, muscles and glands are put together in such a way that you can do a lot of things with them – send semen hurtling toward an egg, feel sexual pleasure and have an orgasm for fun, give pleasure, urinate, and produce hormones that your body needs (mostly to do all of the things just mentioned, along with growing a beard and having generally more muscle mass than women).

Your sex organs and all of the parts of your body that are related to them are fascinating in the way they're assembled and the way that they work.

The Penis

Your penis is the most recognized part of your grouping of sexual organs. It consists of the head (sometimes called the glans), the corona, frenum and urethral meatus, and finally the shaft. Uncircumcised men will also have a foreskin.

So, starting at the tip of your organ, you'll find the urethral meatus. This is the opening where urine and semen come out, and it's located towards the middle of the head. I say "towards" because if you are looking for it to be perfectly centered, you might find that it isn't perfectly centered. Often it is, sometimes it's not – don't worry about it.

The ridge that runs all the way around the bottom of your head is called the corona, and just below the underside of the corona, where it looks like the ridge is coming together, is the frenum – it's that small piece of skin, which for some is extremely sensitive.

Speaking of sensitive, the head is also very sensitive and if you're uncircumcised, your foreskin will most likely be pretty sensitive, too.

The shaft is the part that worries most men when it comes to size – worrying that it's not big enough, as in long or thick enough or both. The shaft looks wrinkly, with a skin color that may be slightly darker than the rest of your skin when you're flaccid. When the shaft is erect, it has bulging veins, and may turn dark red, purple or bluish (the change and variation of color is normal).

If you're not circumcised, you'll also have a foreskin, which I already mentioned can be very sensitive. Foreskin is extra skin that covers the head of your penis when it isn't erect. All men are born with foreskin, but it's become common practice to have it removed in infancy for medical, social or religious reasons.

Some of the medical reasons for circumcision are to help protect against urinary tract infections, prevention of penile cancer, to lower the risk of sexually transmitted diseases, and to prevent a tightening of the foreskin (called phimosis), which essentially closes the penis.

Now that we're all familiar with the outside of the penis, let's see what's inside!

If you've always wondered where all that blood goes when you get an erection, I'm going to clue you in. It's the corpus cavernosum and the corpus spongiosum. These two parts of the penis are spongy areas of soft tissue that fill up with blood, making your organ hard.

And both the corpus cavernosum and the corpus spongiosum extend a little ways into your body, which accounts for your penis becoming erect and standing at attention when filled with blood. These areas will be key in your penis enlargement program.

The urethra is the tube that runs from the tip of your penis to other organs including your bladder and the prostate, and that allows both semen and urine to leave your body through the urethral meatus.

The Testicles

Let's turn our attention to the testicles. Yes, I know you're not looking to making your testicles bigger, but stay with me.

Your testicles, or testes, are enclosed in a sack of muscle-lined skin called the scrotum. This sack hangs just behind and below the penis, and serves as a nice way to protect your testes and keep them from just dangling everywhere.

You've experienced the muscle action of your scrotum when you've jumped into a cold lake or a cold shower. That sack tightens up and draws your testicles in to protect them and keep them warm. Because your testicles are where sperm are manufactured, a lukewarm temperature is best for them – not too hot and not too cold.

Your testicles serve a couple of important functions. First, they produce testosterone, which is the male sex hormone. Second, as mentioned earlier, they produce sperm, which are essential to reproduction.

Each testicle has a small gland sitting on top of it, called the epididymis. That's where your sperm hang out until they're mature.

The vas deferens are the little tubes that take the sperm out of the epididymis, on their way to the prostate gland to be mixed with fluids and then to their final goal of being ejaculated through the urethra.

Just a quick note about your prostate gland – this small, walnut sized gland stores and secretes about a third of the fluid that is expelled from your body when you ejaculate. The prostate also surrounds the urethra. Prostates troubles usually appear in the form of an enlarged prostate. Enlargements of the prostate whether benign or cancerous, can cause problems with getting an erection.

The Pubococcygeus Muscle

The last part of male sexual anatomy that I want to point out to you is the pubococcygeus muscle, also known as the PC muscle. This muscle is going to play a starring role in your program to enhance what you've got and to use it for the enjoyment of not only yourself, but also your partner.

The pubococcygeus muscle is something that both men and women have. It's the muscle that forms your pelvic floor and supports the organs in your pelvic area. Exercising the PC muscle is going to be a part of your program for increasing the size of your penis. It also plays a part in inhibiting premature ejaculation, and in building strong erections and sexual stamina.

The PC muscle is also important for women. It's the muscle that helps her keep her vaginal area firm and tight, so a smart girl will exercise the PC muscle regularly, just as you should.

CHAPTER 3: AVERAGE OR BIGGER – WHICH IS REALLY BETTER?

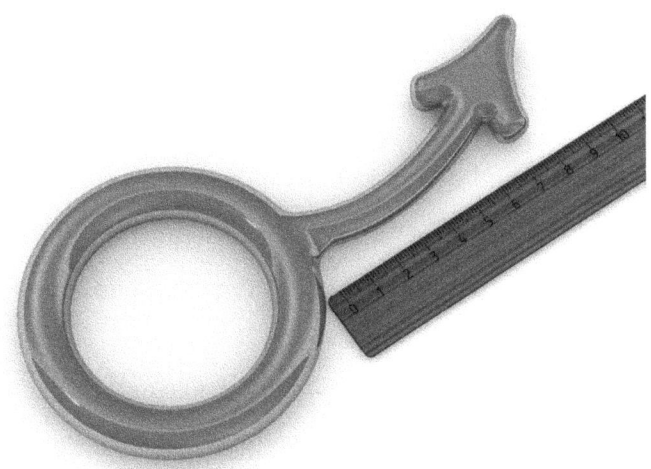

According to research performed in a laboratory setting, average penis size is as follows:

- Length of a flaccid (not erect) penis: 3.4 inches (8.6 cm) to 3.7 inches (9.3 cm)
- Length of an erect penis: 5.1 inches (12.9 cm) to 5.7 inches (14.5 cm)
- Girth of erect penis: 3.5 inches (8.8 cm) to 3.9 inches (10 cm)

Have You Measured Your Penis Yet?

You may not have even measured your penis yet – so you're just guessing about your size. Until you measure, you won't truly know. Many men are shocked when they find that their penis falls within normal range. It's possible that yours does, too.

Part of the trouble is that when you're looking down at your penis, you're not seeing it at the same angle that you would see another man's penis, in the locker room, for example. It's always going to look smaller from the angle you see it from.

And if you're comparing your penis to what you might see in erotic or pornographic material, you have to remember that camera angles, lighting and probably shaving of pubic hair will make a penis appear larger.

Plus, the size of partners in erotic material and films is often very small and petite, and actors in porn movies are often chosen for the fact that they do have larger than normal penises.

So, before you berate yourself for your tiny little penis, do a reality check.

If you seriously do have a penis that falls below the average measurements, or if you are in the average category and still think you want to increase your penis size, then by all means, proceed.

The bottom line is that you need to feel confident about what you've got. Part of that can be accomplished by a good dose of reality. Part will come from developing confidence in other areas and part will happen as you see that your member is getting larger.

The "Big" Questions

So, is bigger really better? The answer to that question depends on a lot of variables.

Here is a list of questions you should ask yourself so you can decide if bigger really is going to be better for you:

1. What are the negative effects of my current penis size on my life?

2. What results do I expect from increasing my penis size? Your expectations could include a more satisfied partner, feeling better about yourself, feeling more masculine, just being able to see it better, feeling like there is something of substance there, etc.
3. Does my partner seem unsatisfied with our sex life? Have we talked about why?
4. Will I feel more sexually satisfied when my penis is larger? Why?
5. Is having a small penis affecting my ability to approach women for dates? Are there other factors?
6. How much length and/or girth do I want to add? Remember that you can aim for King Kong, but be realistic!

- Current length flaccid:
- Goal length flaccid:

- Current length erect:
- Goal length erect:

- Current girth erect:
- Goal girth erect:

7. Is my self-confidence lower because my penis size isn't up to par? Any other reasons?

After you've taken some time to think about and answer these questions, you can decide if bigger is really going to be better for you and then go on with doing something about it.

There is nothing wrong with wanting to increase the size of your penis. If it's going to help your sex life and your self-confidence, then go for it!

Now, before we move on, let's talk about two issues – one is penis shrinkage and the other is masturbation.

Men get pretty upset, and rightfully so, when they notice that their flaccid penis seems to shrink up when they've been exercising. Some men report that strenuous exercise makes their penis and testicles shrivel up and seem to retract right into their groin!

If you run into this problem, don't let it keep you from exercise. This is a very normal reaction in some men, and your penis and testicles will eventually relax back into place and to their normal size. A warm shower can help with this, and a good dose of patience.

Finally, let's discuss masturbation for a moment. Masturbation happens, and most men do it fairly often. Teenaged boys do it a lot! There is a myth that masturbating will make your penis smaller. This is a myth, and only a myth. If you want to masturbate, then do it and don't worry about it.

Chapter 4: Does Size Matter to Women?

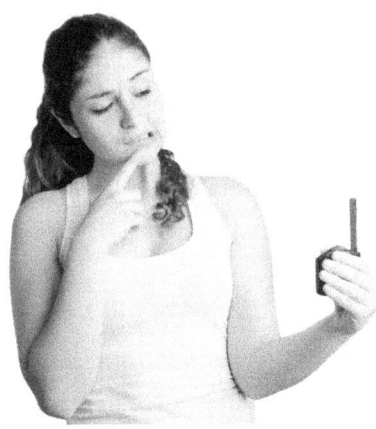

It's good, when you're in the middle of devising your plan for getting an organ the size you want, to remember that you might have a wife or girlfriend who is quite interested in your penis size as well.

And if you don't currently have a sexual partner, you're probably thinking about the prospect of getting one aren't you? The assumption is that women always want a great big penis on their man.

Is that assumption correct?

That question doesn't have a single yes or no answer.

One thing you need to understand about female anatomy is that the vagina is made to fit to the penis. So regardless of your size, she will stretch (or not, as the case may be) to fit you.

The typical vagina of a woman who has not yet had a child is about three inches, or seven and a half cm, long! Does that surprise you? And women who have had children are still about the same size.

Even when a woman is sexually aroused, her vagina is only about four inches, or ten cm, in length. Pretty much any penis, large or small will fit and fill a vagina!

However, many women do like the feeling of being filled a little more and the feeling of her vaginal opening stretching around an erect penis. And if a penis that is larger than four inches comes along, the vaginal tissues will amazingly stretch to fit (assuming it is introduced gradually).

Do Women Care About Penis Size?

The truth is that yes, most women care about penis size. But it's probably not what you're thinking (or panicking about) right now. Most do care, but most don't care that much. And most aren't looking for some guy with a twelve-inch organ, or the next John Holmes. Some women do like super-big penises, and some find them a bit scary.

Truth is, most women want a guy with a penis that falls within average range, or that is only slightly above the average size.

And almost all women agree that regardless of the size of your organ, what is done with it, and whether or not you can bring them to an orgasm (regardless of if it's a vaginal or clitoral orgasm) during sex, makes a bigger difference.

There is more than one way to give a woman a brain-shattering orgasm, and they don't all involve a penis.

So, you have to know how to use it, no matter what its size. And you have to know about all of the other things you can do to make her happy with your sex life together.

What Women Really Want

I'm going to list for you what women want as far as sex goes (these are generalizations – each woman will have her own preferences which may or may not be the same):

- A man who understands female anatomy and how to handle it for her pleasure.
- A man who knows more than one way to produce an orgasm in his partner.
- A man who is able to keep from ejaculating too quickly.
- A man who knows that different positions and different types of strokes with his penis will produce different sensations.
- A man who pays attention to what is making her happy.
- A man with a penis that has enough length and girth to let her know he's in there, but not so big that it causes her discomfort.

So do all women want a guy with a huge member? No. But, it's true that most women want a man with a penis that is impressive (even if for her, that means average size).

Chapter 5: A Big Penis Doesn't Automatically Mean Great Sex - Bedroom Tips for All Sizes

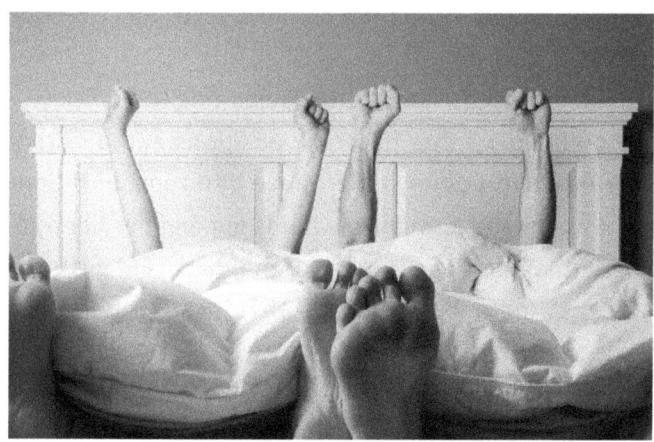

When it comes to sex, penis size isn't as important as you think. There are many aspects to how you perform in the bedroom and intercourse is only one part of the action.

When you take the focus off of your penis size you'll find that you can be more relaxed and have a more fulfilling sexual experience. You just need some helpful tips to improve your sex life without changing your penis size.

Ooze Confidence in the Bedroom

Confidence is a true aphrodisiac in the bedroom. When you exude self-assurance you can take the focus off of size and more on performance. You don't need to bring up your concerns about penis size before you begin a sexual relationship.

There's no need to make an issue out of something that insignificant to most women. Instead, develop sexual techniques that you feel confident about so that you're not worried about your penis.

When it is time for intercourse, you'll find in most cases that you're more than adequate – especially if you follow the rest of the advice in this section.

Listen to Her

One of the most important things you can do in bed is to listen to your partner. Pay attention to what she likes and what isn't working for her. In the actual moment, listen for moaning sounds and for changes in her breathing.

You can also pay attention to the way she's moving her body. Take a mental note of those things that seem to really turn her on. And when you're not in the bedroom, be willing to discuss sex.

You don't need to have a long discussion, but you can ask if there's anything she'd like that you haven't done. Being willing to try new things can help you to have a more satisfying sex life.

Make Her Feel Like a Queen

When you treat a woman well outside the bedroom, you're likely to get a better response in the bedroom. Women need to feel emotionally fulfilled in order to feel sexually fulfilled.

If you treat her badly twenty-three hours out of the day and then expect her to warm up to you for sex, you're not likely to have a good experience – and she definitely won't. So remember to treat her well all the time and you'll reap the rewards in your sex life.

Foreplay

While men tend to be able to go from 0 to 60 MPH in the bedroom in a second, women need a little time to warm up. Don't forget to add foreplay to your routine. The skin is one of the most important sexual organs.

Some foreplay techniques include:

- Set the mood – music and candles can help to set a relaxing mood that invites sexual pleasure

- Body massage - massage helps muscles to relax and allows you to experience intimate nonsexual touch

- Making out – spend some time passionately kissing to help get in the mood (a lot of people skip this step once they begin having intercourse but you should make it a priority all the time)

- Intimate massage – once you've warmed her up a bit, you can begin adding massage to the breasts and genital areas

- Cover her with kisses – don't rush to intercourse but instead spend time covering her entire body with kisses from head to toe

- Suck on her fingers and toes

These techniques help to build sexual excitement and pleasure before introducing intercourse. She'll be much less focused on the size of your penis when she's feeling so stimulated.

Sexual Massage

When it comes to sexual massage, you'll want to spend time caressing her breasts and massaging her vulva. These are both areas of sexual stimulation.

Try massaging the lips of the vulva – this area is often skipped when men focus solely on the vagina. While the vagina does have many nerve endings near its opening, the labia is rich with nerves that provide sexual pleasure.

It's also important not to ignore the most important area between a woman's legs – the clitoris. This is a small gland just above the vaginal opening that becomes enlarged during sexual excitement.

Gently massaging the clitoris in a circular motion can be so satisfying that it produces orgasms. But there's another surefire way to stimulate this area of the body – oral sex.

Oral Sex

One of the best ways you can provide her with sexual fulfillment is to perform oral sex. In fact, many women will have a better orgasm during oral sex than from intercourse alone.

If you're not providing this particular service, you're definitely missing out on the rewards of sexual stimulation you provide. One of the most common techniques that women enjoy is using your tongue to move in a figure eight pattern around the clitoris.

As you perform oral stimulation, pay attention to your partner to make sure you're hitting the right areas.

Be Gentle

One thing men really need to understand about women's genitals is that they're very sensitive. Unlike the penis that's covered in regular skin, the female genitals don't have the top layer of skin. That makes them much more sensitive.

Don't rub too hard or suck too hard when you're stimulating the labia, clitoris, and vagina. Pay attention to signals from your partner. Different women have different preferences for pressure and stimulation. But always start gently.

Intercourse Doesn't Always Bring Orgasm

One important thing to understand about sexual intercourse is that for women it doesn't always bring on orgasm. In fact, there are many women who cannot experience orgasm from intercourse alone.

That's one reason why penis size isn't as big of a deal as you might think. All the things you do leading up to intercourse and during it make a greater difference than the length and girth of your penis.

Clitoral Stimulation during Intercourse

One way you can help her to achieve climax is to stimulate the clitoris during intercourse. You can do that by gently massaging the clitoris with your finger during intercourse.

You can also add the use of a small vibrator that can be placed on the clitoris during sexual intercourse. This adds the extra stimulation that some women need to achieve intercourse during sex.

Ladies First

One of the best things you can during sex is to exercise enough control to allow her to have an orgasm before you do. If you make that your general goal and guideline you'll find that she feels more fulfilled during sex.

If you happen to have an orgasm before she does, make sure to continue stimulating her until she's able to achieve one as well. Just as men become uncomfortable when they are sexually stimulated without an orgasm, women can feel frustrated by not achieving one.

Introduce Sexual Aids

There are many different products on the market that are available to help enhance your sex life. Adding a vibrator or dildo to your sex life can be fun and add to the experience.

You can also add massage oils, creams that provide stimulation, and other products that can support a satisfying sex life. Don't be afraid to add some of these things if you feel that your sex life needs a boost.

Fantasy Play

Another way to enhance your bedroom experience is to add the element of fantasy. That could include role playing, some mild bondage with furry handcuffs or a scarf, or anything upon which you and your partner can mutually agree.

A little whipped cream and chocolate sauce can go a long way in the bedroom. You can also find games to play in the bedroom that help you to get in the mood and have a great time.

Don't be afraid to laugh and be silly during sex – it doesn't always need to be very serious. Sex is supposed to be fun!

Experiment with Positions

Sometimes people get stuck in a rut when it comes to sexual positions. Don't be afraid to try new positions to help improve stimulation during intercourse.

For a more intimate connection, choose positions that allow you to be face to face and make eye contact. Keep the lights on whenever possible so that you can see each other as this improves intimacy and connection.

That doesn't mean you should never use positions that aren't face to face, but make sure that at least some of your sexual experience allows for that contact.

Focus on the Whole Person

Sex is so much more than the size of your penis. When you focus on the whole person and allow you to relax and feel more confident about your sexual performance.

Chapter 6: Is It Really Possible to Make Your Penis Bigger?

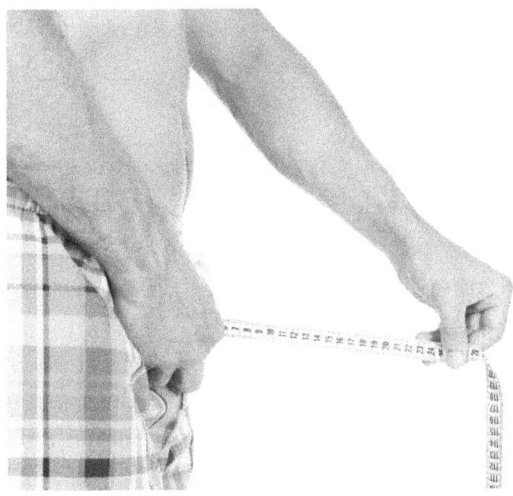

Because you're here reading this, it's safe to say that you've checked out a lot of websites and other information about penis enlargement. I'll bet that you've read that there is no possible way to increase the size of your penis – not with pills, not with pumps, and not with exercises.

And on the other hand, you've read that you can increase the size of your member with any and all of the above listed techniques.

Which Is True?

Because the penis itself is not a muscle, it's true that you can't exercise it and get results the same way as if you were exercising your abs or your biceps. But certain tissues will enlarge gradually when stress is placed on them, or when certain substances stimulate them to grow. This is how penis enlargement works.

So you can make it bigger?

The catch is this: it's not going to happen overnight. Just like losing weight, or working to develop a killer six-pack, or anything else that involves restructuring and re-sculpting your body, enlarging your penis takes time, patience and perseverance.

If you can dedicate yourself to this, you can have a bigger member.

How Long Will It Take?

I'm not going to lie and tell you that you're going to see results in days. It could take several weeks to see improvement, and months to get to your goal, depending on that goal and where you started out. Just like any other exercise routine, you have to do it consistently for a while before you see results.

Bridges are not built in a day, works of art take time to produce, and you'll have to spend time working on your penis before it's exactly the way you want it to be. The good news is that if you start now, you'll be one step, one day closer to your goal!

Chapter 7: Is Penis Enlargement Surgery an Option?

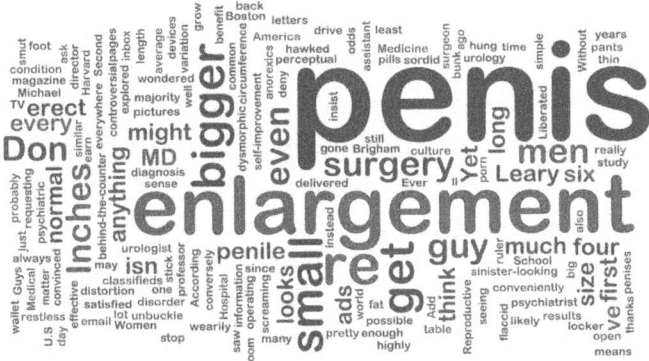

If you're concerned about the size of your penis, you've no doubt considered the idea of penis enlargement surgery. But the idea of going under the knife – especially for such a sensitive area – may seem a little scary.

Before you make such a decision, you should know the facts. You also need to know about home remedies that can help you to have the change you desire without the dangers.

Penis Enlargement Surgery Dangers

Before you make the decision to have a major surgery, it's important to know the facts. First of all, you may have visions of adding a lot of size to your penis through this type of surgery. But the truth is, you'll only add at most, about a half an inch.

For most men this small difference in size will really not make much of a difference when it comes to confidence or pleasuring a partner. And the risks are much greater than the benefits.

The most common procedure to make the penis longer involves cutting the ligament that attaches the penis to your pubic bone. Then, skin is moved from your abdominal area to the penis shaft.

This makes your penis look longer, but it can cause your penis to be unstable when it's erect. In addition to cutting this ligament, sometimes surgeries involve removing fat from the pubic bone to make your penis appear longer.

If you're interested in increasing the girth of your penis, a different procedure is used. The most common way to do this is to transfer fat from one area of your body and inject it into the penis. Unfortunately, this surgery is often disappointing.

That's because the fat is usually reabsorbed by the body and then the increase in width fades away. In addition, the fat can settle in an unbalanced way and actually cause your penis to curve or become uneven.

With any surgery, there's also the possibility that you'll have an infection at the incision point. This can cause pain, swelling, and infection can even result in death in very rare cases.

All in all, penis surgery is painful, expensive, and not very effective. There are much better remedies that you can try at home to help your penis appear larger and to give you more confidence in your ability to please your partner.

Your health and safety are much too important to risk for something that may or may not even work

Exercise is one of the most effective ways to enlarge the penis. It may seem strange because the penis isn't really made of much muscle tissue, but exercise can do a lot to improve your size and performance.

CHAPTER 8: THE PENIS EXERCISE PROGRAM

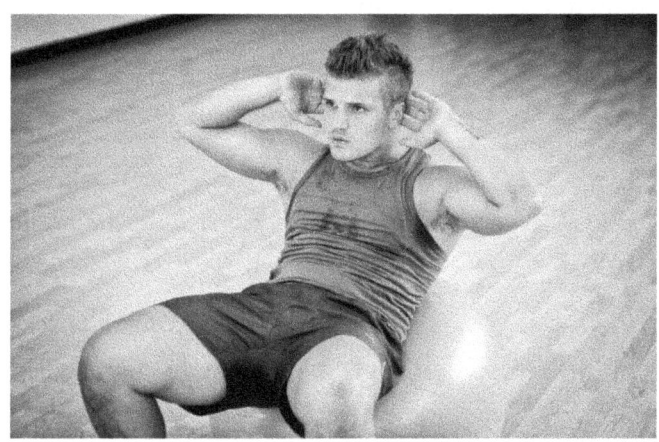

As you may already know, there are several methods that are advertised for enlarging your penis. Exercise is only one of them. But, in many ways it's probably the best. It's completely natural – a hundred percent.

You're not taking any medications and you're not even taking an herbal supplement (yes I know, herbs are natural). The point is that you're only doing exercise – that's it – and it works perfectly by itself.

It's something that benefits the body without adding anything along with it.

As far as using gadgets such as stretchers or weights, yes, these can work, too. But they require you to wear them for hours a day. You might not have time for that, and how convenient is it to attachment something mechanical to your penis and try to have a normal day like that?

So many recommend exercising the penis and PC muscle for the best and most convenient results. That's where the main focus of this section, and actually this book, will be – on developing a solid exercise program that will bring results without having to use anything else.

Start With Some Measurements

Before you begin the exercise program or any type of program to enlarge your penis, you're going to want to take measurements and create a chart to track your growth.

Let's look at the proper way to measure your penis, without cheating.

- The length of your penis is the distance between the tip of your head to where your penis connects to your abdomen (measuring the top of the penis, not the bottom). The circumference of your penis is the distance around the thickest part of the shaft.
- You should measure your member when it is flaccid, and then when it is erect. Make sure that when you're measuring your erect penis that it's as hard as you can possibly get it.
- Length measurements should be done with a ruler, and don't press it into your belly. Just place the ruler against the skin of your abdomen. You want accurate measurements
- When you measure girth, use a fabric tape measure or a piece of yarn or string and wrap it carefully around your penis once, and mark the spot where the measure touches itself. If you're using string or yarn, measure it against a ruler.

You can easily create your own growth chart for recording your measurements either on your computer by using a program such as Excel, or you can do it even more simply by using pen and paper. All you need to do is record your starting date and measurements, and then create spaces to record your progress over two week increments.

If you like, you can use the following information for tracking purposes:

- Start Date
- Flaccid Length
- Erect Length
- Flaccid Girth
- Erect Girth
- +/- Change

Now let's talk about a couple of factors that can affect the way your penis looks, both to you, and others.

The Hair down There

First, consider cutting or completely shaving off your pubic hair. This might sound crazy, but that hair, depending on how much you have down there, can cover up close to an inch of penis when you're observing it from where you are.

It makes it look smaller than it is. As you grow, keep that hair cut close, because whether you think it's cheating or not, it makes a difference in how you look to yourself and to others.

The other reason you want to trim that hair is that when you're doing your penis enlargement exercises, you don't want hair causing discomfort.

Are You Chubby?

Another point that needs to be made very clear is that your level of fitness and your weight is going to have a direct effect on how large or small your sex organ looks. If you have fat hanging around the lower abdominal area, it's going to cause your penis to look smaller.

If you're overweight, why not make this a time to not only get your penis in better shape, but your entire body? Lose some weight through diet and exercise and see what you can do about building your abdominal area and your muscle mass in all parts of your body.

This is automatically going to make you look sexier and will help enhance the look of your penis, too.

It's time to think about actually exercising your penis. There are two things you need to be aware of and always keep in mind when you're doing your enlargement exercise program. They are lubrication and safety.

Lubricate, Lubricate, Lubricate

Your exercise program is going to involve using your hands to manipulate your penis. For some exercises, you will need a good lubricant that will keep the risk of skin irritation and chafing at bay.

You can use a sexual lubricant or a good quality moisturizer. Both of these will probably require reapplication during your exercising, which can be inconvenient. Some men use petroleum jelly, and while this can work well, it's pretty messy. Others like olive oil, which can also be messy. Experiment with what works best for you.

A word of caution: products like shampoo or soap are not good choices for lubricants. They can become very irritating for your skin and cause more trouble than they're worth.

Safety First!

Regardless of whether you're starting a new weight lifting program, or jogging, a new sport, or an exercise program for penis enlargement, you always need to put safety first. Your penis is an important part of your anatomy and you don't want to jeopardize it in any way – you want to enhance it.

If you have any medical conditions that involve your circulatory system or your urinary system, see your doctor before starting this program or before using any type of penis enhancement system or supplement.

As with any type of exercise, a proper warm up is necessary. Pay special attention to warming up before you start on your full-blown workout. If you notice any sores or blisters developing, they could be the result of not properly warming up. You will need to take a few days off to let them heal before starting the program again. Remember to warm up!

If you notice some small, blue spots developing under the penis skin, take a few days off, and use warm wraps (we'll discuss wraps soon) a few times a day. Those blue spots are tiny bruises where some bleeding has occurred, called petechiae. They will disappear in a few days. However, if they seem to get worse, see your doctor immediately.

It's very rare that an exercise program like this would cause any type of problem at all. Be sure to follow all instructions carefully and warm up and cool down properly. If you do this, you'll have a great experience!

Let's Get Started – The Basics

As already mentioned, a warm up is going to be paramount for getting a good workout that is safe, comfortable and that brings some great results, so we'll start with a couple of warm up techniques.

- The first way to warm up is simple: take a warm shower or bath. Five minutes is enough to loosen up connective tissue and draw blood into the penis and improve circulation in the penis and groin area.

- The other way to warm up is to do a Hot Wrap. Take a clean washcloth or hand towel and moisten it with hot water – not scalding, but nice and warm. Wring the towel out and then wrap both your penis and testicles in it.

Leave it for two or three minutes, and then repeat the process of wetting the towel with hot water and wrapping your penis and testicles in it, twice more. When you're finished, dry yourself thoroughly.

Exercise the PC Muscle for a Healthy Prostate and Better Sex!

Did I mention that exercising your PC muscle will give your penis a stronger, more muscular look, too?

Remember in the Male Anatomy chapter where I told you that knowing what the pubococcygeus muscle is and where it is would come in handy later in the book? Well, we're here – this is the place. The PC muscle is going to be an integral part of your penile enhancement program.

The PC muscle is actually a part of both male and female anatomy. In men, this muscle controls semen and urine flow, the firmness of your erections, and also the power behind your ejaculations. Keeping your PC muscle strong is one of the keys to keeping your erections nice and hard, well into your senior years.

The PC muscle, when exercised with Kegel exercises, is also a big help when it comes to controlling orgasms and ejaculations.

And your prostate will thank you for exercising your PC muscle regularly. PC exercise massages the prostate, which helps keep it healthy - and a healthy prostate is a very good thing.

What's a Kegel?

A Kegel exercise is what you're going to do to strengthen your PC muscle. Kegels are easy to do, and here's the best part – you can do them anywhere, and no one will ever know!

To do a Kegel exercise, all you have to do is contract the muscle and then let it relax. That's it. And you can do as many as you want each day. In fact, you should work up to a high number of Kegels every day. Once you learn how, it's not hard to start building that muscle.

You can do Kegels on the way to work, at your desk or work station, waiting in line at the fast food joint, while calling your mother to wish her a happy birthday, and while you're falling asleep at night.

You can stand, sit, or lie down to do Kegels and in fact, it's probably better if you do your exercises in a variety of positions. There are several variations of Kegel exercises that you will learn in this section.

How to Find Your PC Muscle

You know where your PC muscle is, but you might be uncertain of how to make sure you've found it, and not something else. The best way to find the PC muscle is to stop the flow of urine the next time you use the bathroom. When you do that, you'll feel your PC muscle contract.

Now that you've found it, you need to make sure you only contract that muscle when you do your Kegel exercises and leave the surrounding muscles relaxed. The temptation is to contract your abdominals, your thighs and your buttocks, too. Don't do that! Leave them relaxed and concentrate the contraction on your PC muscle.

You now know where it is and how to contract it. Now it's time to exercise it.

The PC Muscle Exercises

Here's where the going gets a little tough. Don't panic, though - building the PC muscle is just like building any other muscle. You do it through repetitions and by increasing intensity as the muscle strengthens.

There are several different ways to work your PC muscle, and all are going to contribute to better, stronger erections, stronger ejaculation, more pleasure for you and your partner, and increased confidence.

Your PC muscles will be worked out during your regular exercise routines, but you should also do PC exercises through your day. They don't all have to be done in one sitting.

Warm It Up

Just like any other muscle, you have to warm up your PC muscle before you start strenuously exercising it. Don't do anything until you've warmed up.

PC warm ups are quick and easy – they are simple contractions – contract and let go, contract and let go, in a steady pace. When you contract, contract as tightly as you can. Then relax all the way.

Do this twelve times per set for three sets, with a short (10 to 15 second) break in between sets. This sounds easy, but when you start out, it might not be. Do what you can, and work up to it. Just remember that before you move on to more advanced moves, you need to be able to get good and warmed up.

Now you're finished warming up your PC muscle and you can move on to PC muscle workouts. There are a few different workouts you can do, and it's best if you rotate them, instead of only doing one or two of the workouts.

PC Workout #1 – Standard Contractions

You'll do standard contractions here – tighten all the way up, and then fully relax the contraction. Your eventual goal will be to do hundreds – literally. Some guys have worked up to a thousand a day (for the days they are doing this particular workout).

Begin by warming up. Once warmed up, work in sets of 25. Take a break of one minute between each set. If you can do ten sets, that's great - especially to begin with. If you work up to forty sets – there's a thousand standard Kegels!

Note that you do not have to do all of these at one time. You can spread your Kegels throughout the day.

PC Workout #2 – Flutters

PC Flutters are much like standard contractions, except you move more quickly. The contractions aren't going to be as tight and sustained, and your relaxation won't be full. This is rapid contracting and relaxing.

You're going for endurance here. You want to see how long you can keep the flutter going. Try to sustain the flutter exercise for one minute, and then rest for one to three minutes. Try to repeat this at least five times.

PC Workout #3 – Flex It and Hold It

The Flex and Hold workout is a bit more advanced, but properly warmed up beginners shouldn't shy away from doing it.

The way you do a flex and hold is to contract the PC muscle tightly, and hold there for a count of ten (longer if possible). This is hard to do, but once you get your muscle to the point where you can successfully do it, you're well on your way to total PC fitness!

Do the Flex and Hold three to four times each day, and allow yourself to relax for one minute between flexes.

PC Workout #4 – Intensity Increases

This is also an advanced PC muscle workout, but don't be afraid to try it. Start by lightly contracting your PC muscle and holding for three seconds. Then contract a bit more and hold again for three seconds.

Now contract it as tightly as you can and hold for another three seconds. Relax by going doing the opposite – relax a little and hold, then relax a bit more and hold, and then finally relax all the way. Rest for thirty seconds and try again.

Work up to ten Intensity Increases a day (you'll do some in your regular workouts and you can do more throughout your day when convenient).

PC Workout #5 – Find the Beat

This is a Kegel workout that can be fun, but it takes some concentration and it can be hard to do. Again, don't let that stop you from trying until you can do it like an expert. This is easiest to do with music – something that has some rhythm variations. Just contract and relax in time to the beat and keep going throughout the song.

The other thing you can do, and this is great when you're driving, is to contract when you hit a marker, like an intersection or when you see a certain colored car, then hold on until your hit another maker, or the light at the intersection turns or something like that.

You have to use your imagination to come up with predetermined "beats" for contractions and relaxations.

PC Workout #6 – The Hanging Towel

This is an interesting and fun way to strengthen your PC muscle. The first thing you need is a full erection. Once you've established that, hang a hand towel over your penis (covering your entire penis).

Now flex the PC muscle and then let it relax. Your penis should move up and down. You won't find this exercise in the regular workout routine, but you can mix it in to your routine for customization, or throw a few towel hangs in a few times a week after your shower.

As you build up some strength and stamina, you can graduate to a larger towel. And because your erect penis is directly involved in this exercise, you're strengthening your PC muscle and also causing your penis to build more tissue due to the gentle pressure the towel is putting on it.

The Work Is Worth the Reward

Kegels are going to be the foundation of your penis enhancement and enlargement exercise program. Do Kegel exercises make your penis bigger? No, they don't – not directly (except for the Hanging Towel exercise).

But all the Kegel exercises are extremely important because exercising your PC muscle means that you're building the foundation for growth, better erections, better control over ejaculation and more sexual power.

You can't build a house without a proper foundation and you can't grow your penis to a bigger size without a proper foundation either. The PC muscle is that foundation. Make it as strong as you possibly can!

Stretch It Out!

Stretching exercises are going to focus on length. You're essentially going to be working on making your sex organ longer – these exercises don't do anything for girth. However, stretching is an integral part of your penis enlargement program, so don't slack on these. They're important!

Stretching your penis can really work to make it longer. The skin and tissue of your penis are not much different than those of other parts of your body. You've seen how people can stretch their earlobes out in the fairly new practice of gauging. And before gauging came along, women's earlobes commonly stretched longer from wearing heavy, dangling earrings.

Another example of how stretching can permanently change the body is The Pa Dong Long Neck people of Thailand. In this culture, extremely long necks are considered beautiful for women, so at the young age of six, metal bands are snapped around girl's necks to gradually stretch them.

Over the years, up to twenty-eight bands may be placed around a woman's neck to lengthen it, and it does work. These are two examples of how body parts can be stretched to longer lengths. The penis is no different.

The stretching exercises that will be outlined here are as effective as lengthening your penis by using weights or a stretcher (which we'll discuss later in this book). However, they are much, much more convenient and safer, too.

Your repertoire of penis stretching exercises is going to consist of combinations of stretching, twirling and slapping. Don't get freaked out. This isn't as crazy as it might sound, and these exercises do produce results by encouraging your penis skin and tissues to lengthen.

You can do your exercises either sitting down or standing. It's your choice.

Let's get started.

The Basic Stretch

This is a very basic exercise, and in fact, it can be looked at as a stretching warm up (although you still must do your basic warm up with a warm, wet towel, a warm bath or shower first).

The basic stretch goes like this: Make an OK sign with your fingers – your thumb and index finger meet, forming a circle, and your other three fingers are up.

With your other hand, hold your penis at the base to stabilize it.

Now encircle your flaccid penis, just below the head, with your OK sign, palm facing away from you. Gently, but firmly, pull outward, and then relax the penis back inward. Pull out, relax in.

Continue this exercise for ten repetitions and then repeat the process with your other hand.

Dry Milking

Dry milking has some advantages. For one, you don't use any lubricants, which can be messy. It can also be done just about anywhere (as long as you have privacy), again because you don't have to mess around with lubricants. You still need to do a warm up though.

Start with a partial erection, as with wet milking.

Now, beginning at the base of your penis, firmly grip yourself with the OK sign and without sliding your fingers over the skin, move the

OK sign towards the head, but not all the way to the head. Loosen your grip, and then move back to the base.

Work the base area in this manner for a while, and then work the middle of the shaft in the same manner.

If you experience any soreness or discomfort, take a day off from dry milking.

As with wet milking, you don't want to get a full erection.

Wet Milking

Let's go through the steps of wet milking one by one:

First, warm up. Don't skip this step because your penis needs this to ready itself or jelqing. (Jelqing is a form of repetitive penile massage performed on a semi-tumescent penis that, over time, will increase the length and girth of the penis). If you don't warm up, you risk injuring yourself. It's that simple.

Next, use a good amount of lubricant on your penis to develop a partial erection. Keep it to a maximum of sixty percent erect.

Now, grasp the base of your penis with one hand making the OK sign. Your palms can face either away or toward you – whichever is most comfortable. Your grip should be gentle, but firm. Now draw that hand all the way to the bottom of the head.

At this point, use your other hand to form an OK sign and do the same thing, as you release the grip of the first hand.

As the second hand reaches the head, you will grasp your penis again in the same manner and "milk" your penis down to the head.

Repeat this process in a rhythmic motion, using both hands and applying fresh lubricant as needed.

The beginning goal is to do between two and three-hundred jelq strokes a day with a medium firm grip for the first week that you jelq. You will work upward to a stronger grip over the upcoming weeks (we'll get to that soon).

When you've finished wet milking, cool down and encourage good circulation by doing side to side slaps (twenty to thirty on each side).

Jelqing should be done five days a week

Remember, you need to do this while only partially erect. If you start to get a full erection, squeeze harder to suppress the erection or stop and wait until you are at fifty to sixty percent erect.

Jelqing is basically an exercise that teaches you self-control and that works to expand the tissues of your penis by forcing more blood into them.

Jelqing for Length and Girth

The Jelq exercise is said to have origins in the Middle East, with Europeans making it a popular technique for enlarging the penis.

Jelqing is a method that is based on the idea that the corpus cavernosum and spongiosum can be made larger, giving them the ability to hold more blood when the penis is erect. Jelqing, sometimes called milking the penis, is a technique that pushes blood into the penis, holds it there and then pushes more blood into the penis, causing it to expand to a larger size that it had originally been.

An illustration of how this works would be to fill a balloon halfway with water and then to clamp the balloon, pushing the water further to the end. Continuing to push this water further to the end causes the rubber to expand even more.

This is like what happens with jelqing. If you were to add even more water to the balloon, and push it closer to the end, the balloon would continue to expand and enlarge. This is how jelqing works on your member.

A daily jelqing workout takes between fifteen and thirty minutes, and begins with your basic warm up of a warm shower or bath, or wrapping with warm, moist towels. This prepares your penis for jelqing and other exercises by stimulating blood flow to the penis.

Jelqing should be done only on a semi-erect penis, not an erect one, and should not cause ejaculation. "Wet milking" and "dry milking" are the two main types of jelqing, and both are effective in bringing about permanent enlargement.

We'll start with the wet milking technique. This is where a good lubricant will come in handy – in fact, it's a necessity, so if you haven't got one yet, you need to get one now. Please revisit the section on lubricants, and remember, don't use soap or shampoo!

The Tao Technique of Jelqing

The Tao technique focuses solely on increasing the size of your head and can be used in combination with both wet and dry milking.

With the Tao method, you will use a wet milking technique, but you will concentrate on working more slowly and gently, and pushing the blood into your penis head and holding that pressure for a sustained period of time. This will create a more pronounced mushroom, bell or helmet shaped head.

Begin by lubricating your penis and using the OK sign to milk your organ and push more blood through it and to the end. Using your fingers, work the blood into the head and hold it there for ten seconds. You can squeeze the shaft to help make the head engorge.

Once the head is hard, release and repeat.

With the Tao method, you should limit your time to a maximum of ten minutes.

Pulling and Slapping

Now this sounds rather violent! But again, it's just a part of the penis stretching exercise routine.

Start by grasping your flaccid penis close to the base. Now, use your OK sign to hold your penis just below the head, palm facing away, and pull outward for twenty to thirty seconds.

Next, just by holding your organ at the base, slap it twenty times to one side, hitting your leg, and then twenty times to the other side, again hitting the leg.

Complete the exercise by pulling up and outward again by using your OK sign just below the head. Hold for twenty seconds.

Stretching and Twirling

Sounds like an interpretive dance style, doesn't it - Stretching and Twirling? Well, it's really a type of penis stretching exercise where you stretch and then sort of swing your penis clockwise and then counter-clockwise.

Get comfortable and get a grip on your penis as described for the basic stretch exercise, with either of your hands. Now, while holding a gentle, but firm stretch, pull slightly toward the side of your hand (right or left), and twirl (not twist – there's a difference!) your member clockwise ten times, then counter-clockwise ten times.

Repeat the process with the opposite hand and side.

Combined Pull, Twirl and Slap

This is a bit advanced, and takes some concentration.

Begin by using your OK sign to pull outward and hold for several seconds. Make sure the palm of your hand is facing away from you.

Now hold your penis by the base and with your OK sign in place, twirl your penis clockwise five times and then counter clockwise five times.

Pull outward again, and then twirl again in the same way as mentioned above. Do this entire sequence five times.

Now pull outward for several seconds and do twenty slaps on each side.

Finish by pulling up and outward for thirty seconds.

Sometimes all of this handling and movement causes a feeling of arousal. Don't worry about it, just stop exercising and give your erection a chance to subside. Then begin where you left off.

Cool It Down!

Now that you've exercised your penis, you have to cool it down. You can't just put it in your pants and forget it until next time.

There are a few different ways to cool down – all are meant to encourage blood flow and good circulation. You can:

- Do some slaps – let it get flaccid first.
- Wait until it's completely flaccid and then give it a good massage. This isn't meant to start an erection, though.
- Take a nice warm shower or bath, or wrap your penis and testicles with a nice, warm, moist towel.
- Exercising your penis puts a fair amount of stress on it. Give it a chance to relax now.

CHAPTER 9: CREATE AN EXERCISE SCHEDULE FOR YOUR PENIS

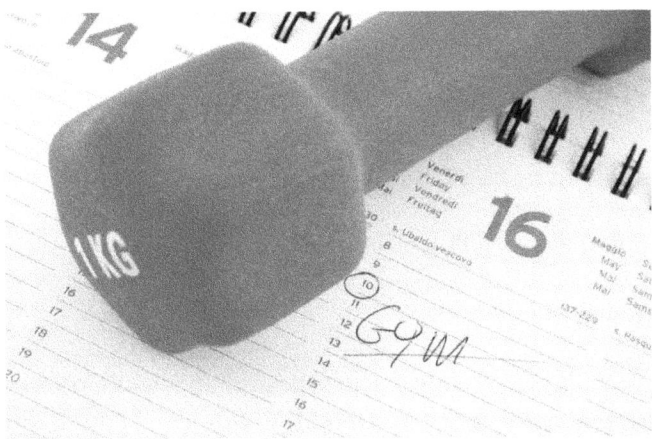

Here's where the rubber meets the road. It's time to get started and to keep a schedule that introduces your penis and PC muscle to enhancement exercises and then increases the intensity of your workouts, and your results over the period of several weeks.

You're going to be spending time five days a week exercising your penis and your PC muscle. It's going to take time out of your day – you need to commit yourself to that right now because if you slack off because you're tired, or you don't want to miss your favorite TV show or some other lame excuse, the only person you're hurting is yourself.

Schedule time each week for this program. On the days you're scheduled to exercise, plan for it – just like you would set aside time to go to the gym or to study for a class if you're a student, or to spend with your friends or family. You might have to get up a bit earlier, or sacrifice some couch potato time. As the old Nike ads say, Just Do It!

Your first two weeks are going to start out fairly easy, but don't let that fool you – you'll be getting a good workout! You just can't jump into to doing an advanced workout yet – you don't want to injure yourself!

First Couple of Weeks

Plan to exercise five days per week. You can do three on, one off, two on, one off, or all five days in a row with two off. It's up to you. But you need to be consistent about exercising five days per week.

Your first few weeks will look like this:

1. Warm up

Use the techniques already discussed. Don't neglect a proper warm up! This should take about five minutes.

2. PC muscle exercises

Even though you may be doing PC muscle exercises in a multitude of places at different times during your day, you should do some as part of your "formal workout," too.

As part of this workout, you should do standard contractions. You'll spend two to five minutes on this. Do take some time to do the PC muscle warm up. This is just lighter intensity contractions, and shouldn't take more than a couple minutes.

3. Stretch exercises

You should plan on doing a variety of stretching exercises for about ten minutes each workout. Look at the stretching exercise section and plan to either do some of each during your workout, or rotate the type of stretching exercise you do throughout the week.

4. Break for circulation

After stretching, spend one minute either massaging your penis (flaccid) or slapping it to get the blood moving around.

5. Jelqing (wet milking)

You can spend up to ten minutes jelqing, and should spend at least five minutes doing this exercise.

6. Cool down

Your cool down will take about five minutes.

There you have it! You'll spend around thirty minutes per workout. If you're consistent, you'll begin to see small changes even by the end of the first week. Your penis probably won't be larger, but your erections and your self-control when it comes to ejaculation will already be improved!

Weeks Three through Six – Moving On Up!

It's time to intensify things a bit. You'll still be spending about thirty minutes, five days a week on exercising your penis and PC muscle, but it's time to get tougher with yourself.

1. Warm Up – This should go without saying. Every workout you ever do has to start with a good warm up.
2. PC Muscle Exercises – Here's where things are going to get a little tougher.
   - Warm up with some quick and light contractions.
   - Start with standard contractions. Do twenty repetitions.
   - Next, do three sets of Flex and Hold contractions – eight contractions each set.
   - Finish with one minute of Flutters
3. Continue with practicing a variety of stretching exercises for ten minutes.

4. Take a one-minute break for circulation. Massage or slap your penis against your legs.
5. Do a minimum of seven minutes of jelqing, up to a maximum of 10 minutes.
6. Cool down.
7. Three times per week, try dry milking in addition to wet milking. Don't do your dry milking during your regular workout. You can do it in the evening at bedtime or another convenient time. Spend between five and ten minutes dry milking.

Note: You should be doing PC muscle exercises throughout your day – not just during your regular workout. Try some of the more advanced PC contractions.

The Halfway Mark – You're on Your Way!

You may already be noticing some improvements. Even if they are small, you know you're on the right track! Don't lose your momentum now!

It's time to step things up! Your workout is going to be slightly longer now – the extra time and intensity will be well worth it!

1. Warm up thoroughly.
2. Get that PC muscle in shape! You should be doing PC exercises during your workouts, and you should also be doing them randomly throughout your day. Remember that you can't do too many of these! What you're getting in your workout is great, but do extra PC exercises to boot.
    - Start with a quick PC warm up and then do standard contractions. Do forty repetitions.
    - Now, do some Intensity Increases. These are hard, but you've been working your PC muscle a lot, so it should be up for the challenge! Do a minimum of five and work up to ten over these weeks (you don't have to do all ten during this workout, but you should make a point to do at least

ten per day now).
- Finish with two minutes of sustained Flutters.
3. Over the first few weeks, you've been doing any variety of stretching exercises for ten minutes each session. Now we're going to get more specific. You are going to do the Combined Pull, Twirl and Slap exercise pretty much exclusively. It incorporates all the stretching exercises into on. Do this combination exercise five times – the entire sequence.
4. You'll need a circulation break now. Give your penis a one-minute massage to encourage blood flow and good circulation.
5. You can choose either wet milking or dry milking for your exercise now. If you are wet milking, increase your grip to slightly firmer than what you've been doing. From here on out, jelq with a firmer grip (but don't hurt yourself!) Do this for ten minutes.
6. Cool down.

By now, you will have noticed that your penis is longer and has more girth. You will also have noticed that your erections are much, much stronger and that you have more stamina along with better control over your ejaculations.

You probably aren't however, at you goal length and girth. This takes time, just like all good things. What you need to do now is keep going. You can continue with this workout, and even add your own variations to keep it interesting.

Tired of doing certain PC muscle exercises? Don't forget the Hanging Towel and Find the Beat exercises. They're both great for your PC muscle!

You can do the Tao method of jelqing sometimes if you like – remember this works especially well for developing the head of your penis.

The key is to keep exercising consistently, and don't slack off. Keep up with your two week measurements, too. Don't measure yourself every day! This is a terrible idea because you won't see daily changes and you'll get discouraged. When you measure every two weeks, you've given yourself enough time to make more positive impact on your growth, and you'll feel excited and encouraged to keep going!

Let's talk about some specialized exercise programs now.

The Quickie

Now it's not what you're thinking! But even though you should be spending a half hour to around forty-five minutes on your workouts, there may be days when you honestly don't have that kind of time.

Here's what you do:

1. Warm up and do PC muscle exercises together. This means that while you're in the shower getting your genital region all warmed up, you're doing standard contractions, Flex and Hold, Intensity Increases or Flutters in combination. You can also do PC exercises if you're warming up with a warm wrap.

2. Dry milk – if you're in a hurry, forget wet milking – it's too messy and requires clean up depending on the lubricant you use. Do five minutes of dry milking.

3. Do three Combined Pull, Twirl and Slap exercise sequences

4. Finish with one minute of massage.

There you go – you've spent about fifteen minutes, maximum.

While doing a quick workout is fine on occasion, this should not be your regular way of exercising, because it's not as effective. It's like a one-mile walk vs. a three-mile walk. Both are very good for your health, but that extra two miles is going to make a bigger difference in the long run. Still if you're pressed for time, or tired, one mile will help your fitness.

CHAPTER 10: EXERCISE CAN INCREASE SIZE AND CORRECT OTHER ISSUES

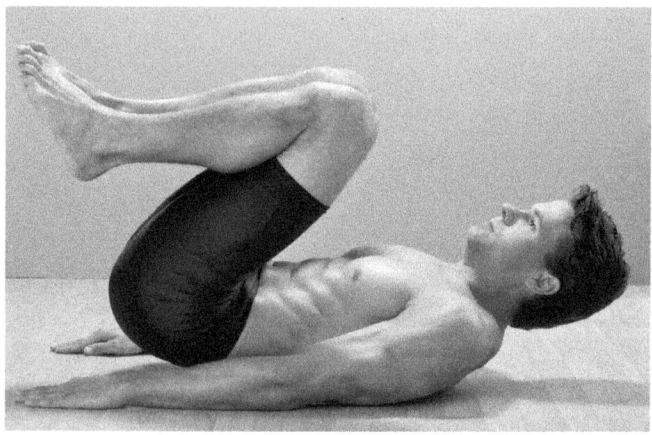

It's already been mentioned that some of the exercises taught in this book can help immensely with ejaculation control, but other issues can be corrected with exercise, too.

Some men have a penis that curves slightly to the left or right, or even up or downward – exercise can help!

For men that simply cannot always get an erection, or a quality erection, exercise can help.

Let's take each issue one by one.

Premature Ejaculation

This, like having a smallish penis, is not something that men want to have to deal with, and yet, it happens. Sometimes, it is nearly impossible to keep from losing your load way too early. It's embarrassing, but it's also something that can be cured.

Currently, there are no prescription medications that work specifically for premature ejaculation. However, doctors sometimes prescribe certain antidepressants or topical creams that reduce sensation to help slow the ejaculation response down. While these can help, they are not a cure, and all medications come with side effects.

If you like the idea of using a topical cream, but without a prescription, you can find creams and sprays that make your penis less sensitive online and at shops that sell erotic materials and toys. These can be very helpful.

Some herbal remedies are said to help with premature ejaculation – dodder seed is one. We'll talk about herbs soon.

And often doctors and therapists will recommend that you masturbate an hour or so before sex, so that you won't ejaculate as quickly when you're with your partner. This is actually a very good idea.

Other things you can do to help with this issue are strengthen the PC muscle (and you're already doing that, right?), and learn self-control.

Learning self-control really isn't that hard to do, and in fact, it can be pretty fun! Simply masturbate more – a lot more! You should masturbate once a day in fact. During your masturbation sessions, teach yourself to stop and hold back when you start to feel that you're getting close to ejaculating.

At first, it might seem hard, but keep practicing! When you feel that sensation, stop masturbating, and squeeze the base of your penis (not too hard!). At the same time, contract your PC muscle. Hold back the feeling. When it begins to subside, start masturbating again, and then hold back. Do this several times. You're training yourself to not ejaculate so quickly!

A Curved Penis

A curved penis is the source of much distress for men. Having a severely curved penis (Peyronie's disease) isn't uncommon, and can be usually be cured without surgical intervention.

Peyronie's disease is a curvature that is so pronounced that intercourse is impossible and erections are often painful. If you have this problem, see your doctor, and don't be embarrassed – Peyronie's really is not uncommon – doctors have seen it before and know how to treat it.

Now, if your penis is just slightly curved, you needn't fear that you have a disease that needs medical treatment (although if it will help, see your doctor to be sure). Often, in this case, these slight curvatures can be fixed with regular exercise.

1. When you are practicing your basic stretching exercise, do about half of the strokes in the opposite direction of the curve. So if you curve to the left, simply stroke right, against the direction of the curve, half the time. Be gentle when you're doing this.
2. You can also work on straightening your curve when you're wet milking. Do the exercise as normally recommended, but for every eight normal strokes, do two that go against the curve.
3. Never try to bend or force the curve to straighten! Use gentle pressure only.

Impotence

Impotence is generally thought of as the result of aging. But young men can suffer from impotence, and older men can have a fantastic sex life well into their golden years!

Impotence can be caused by the complications of getting older, but certain medications, drug use, alcohol abuse, smoking and certain health conditions can also make it difficult to get and maintain an erection.

There are some effective prescription drugs available to help achieve and maintain and erection (we'll talk about the in a later chapter. But it is a heartening and happy fact that exercising the PC muscle will help to solve impotence!

Because the PC muscle is so important to penis health and healthy erections, it is the foundation of curing impotence. If you're already doing the workout for enlargement, you're getting a good PC muscle workout. If you're not doing the enlargement workout, learn the PC muscle exercises and do them! They will help.

Note about erectile dysfunction: Sometimes the inability to get an erection is caused by an underlying illness. You should consult with your doctor to rule out any health problems that could be causing this. It's probably as simple as needing to strengthen your PC muscle, and possibly making some changes in your habits, but it's best to be sure.

Now you have a full exercise program for enlarging your penis, both by length and girth and also for solving some other pesky penis problems. We'll move on now to take a look at other penis enhancement and enlargement techniques.

You might choose to use one of them, which is fine, but if you do, you should seriously consider still doing the workouts. A strong PC muscle is great for prostate health, not to mention your sex life. And using exercise to enlarge your penis is the most cost-effective, convenient and natural way.

CHAPTER 11: DO PILLS, SUPPLEMENTS, AND GADGETS WORK?

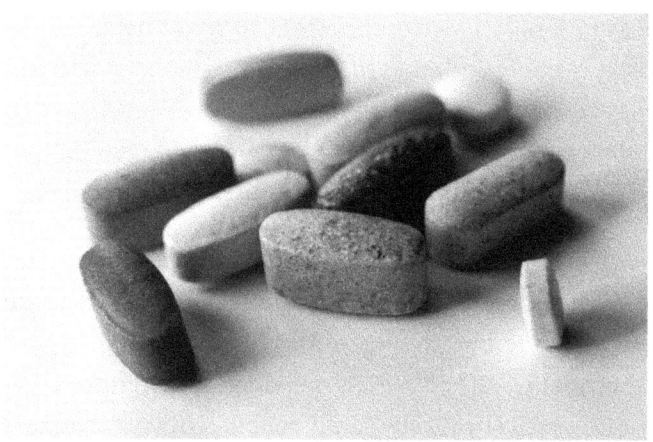

There are a couple of different areas where pills, medications, supplements and gadgets such as pumps are used for male enhancement. Enlargement is one area, but let's not forget the medications (both prescription and over the counter) that help men to get and keep an erection, and those that are used to make men "hornier."

Even though you primarily bought this book looking for information on how to grow your penis to a larger, more appreciable size, let's not forget that stamina, horniness and the ability to hold on for a goodly amount of time before ejaculating are all things that will add to your prowess and masculinity.

You can have the biggest organ in the world, but if you're not horny, or don't have staying power, that big penis is only going to be there for looks. And if you can't "get it up" in the first place, well, that's not much fun, is it?

Some of these enhancement inducers work, some don't. Some will work well for one man, and not so well for another. When it comes to prescription medications, your doctor will help you decide which is going to work best for you, and some experimentation might be necessary to see which is best.

It's time to look at all those pills and things and figure out what they're good for, if they work, and what they might do to, and for you.

Prescription Drugs

Viagra, Levitra and Cialis are all prescriptions medications that won't help you get a bigger organ, but they can help you get an erection if you're having trouble in that area (erectile dysfunction). They don't increase your desire to have sex either, but make it possible to act on that desire.

These drugs are for helping to achieve and sustain an erection. You may not have any problems with this today, but consider the following statistics:

- One out of 10 men have some form of erectile dysfunction.
- The likelihood of having erectile problems increases with age, but relatively young men may suffer from erectile dysfunction. By the age of forty, thirty-nine percent of men have problems with getting and keeping erection.
- Diabetics and smokers have a higher risk of developing erectile dysfunction, as do men who have high levels of stress in their lives, low testosterone levels or who abuse alcohol or take certain types of medications.

No one wants to talk about not being able to get an erection and keep it going, but the reality is that many men suffer from this problem. If you add it to a small penis issue, you've really got a tough situation. The good news is that it can be resolved, so don't give up!

Prescription drugs that help with erectile dysfunction work by blocking PDE5, a chemical that will cause an erection to subside. While they do work well, you can strongly enhance your ability to get and keep an erection by doing PC exercises and making some healthy lifestyle changes, such as quitting smoking.

Prescription medications for erectile dysfunction do come with side effects such as flushing, headache, upset stomach and stuffy or runny nose. Muscle aches, back pain and temporary vision changes have also been reported.

There are some rare, but serious side effects to these medications as well, including vision loss, hearing loss and erections that don't subside on their own after a few hours – these serious side effects should immediately be reported to your doctor.

Drugs for erectile dysfunction can also interact with other drugs and shouldn't be used if you have certain medical conditions.

One last note about erectile dysfunction: you should consult with your doctor to rule out any underlying illness that may be causing your problem.

Natural Pills and Supplements

Before we talk about supplements for penis enlargement, you need to know that these haven't been evaluated by the FDA or any governing body that looks after such things as drugs. This doesn't mean that they won't work, or that they are harmful. All it means is that the FDA hasn't checked them out and given their own seal of approval as a drug that works.

As you probably already know, whether you're using a medication prescribed by a doctor, or taking a natural supplement, there are always risks of side effects and interactions with drugs, so you should always use due caution.

Now that we've gotten past all that, let's talk about penis enlargement pills.

You are familiar with the way your penis is built, right? You know about the corpus cavernosum and the corpus spongiosum. These are the chambers in your penis that fill with blood when you're aroused. Blood fills your penis to the maximum amount it's able to hold when you're fully excited and that's what gives you an erection.

This is a scientific fact. It's also a fact that if the underlying tissue grows, your skin will grow to accommodate it. So the method behind any form of penis enlargement is to get the corpus cavernosum and spongiosum to grow.

When you do that, your penis will be larger when flaccid, but also larger when erect because there is more room for blood to fill it.

Penis enhancement pills use natural substances to stimulate the growth of the soft tissue that make up these two areas of your penis. The also use substances such as herbs to help you feel more aroused and sensitive and give you more energy and staying power.

Which Natural Substances Will You Find in Penis Enhancement Pills?

Different pills will have their own unique mixtures of ingredients, so I've created a list of common ingredients that you can find in male enhancement supplements, along with what their function is.

- L-arginine – This naturally occurring amino acid helps to relax and open up blood vessels, by forming nitric oxide in the body. Nitric oxide expands your blood vessels allowing oxygen-rich blood and nutrients to rich every organ. L-arginine also

stimulates the release of growth hormones, and increases ejaculatory volume and orgasm intensity.
- Dodder Seed (also called Tu su zi or semen cuscutae) – Dodder seed helps strengthen your urogenital functions and is commonly used to treat lack of libido, frequent urination, premature ejaculation and impotence. In traditional Chinese medicine, it is considered to be an aphrodisiac.
- Gingko (Folium ginkgoidis) – Ginkgo leaf extract is used to enhance blood circulation and increase blood flow to the penis.
- Yin yang huo (Herba epimdii) – Yin yang huo increases hormonal secretions, sperm count and semen density.
- Yohimbe (Corynanthe yohimbea) – Yohimbe is used as an aphrodisiac.
- Damiana (Turnera aphrodisiaca) – Damiana has a reputation for increasing sexual stamina, improving erectile function and enhancing orgasms.
- Puncture Vine (Tribulus terrestris) – This herb is reported to increase the level of testosterone in the body, enhance libido, and improve stamina.
- Epimedium Leaf (Epimedium sagittatum) – Also known as Horny Goat Weed, epimedium leaf has been known and used for years as a libido booster. Epimedium has also been found to increase blood flow to the penis, much in the same way that prescription medications for erectile dysfunction do. Horny goat weed also helps to increase sensation and restore sexual power.
- Asian Red Ginseng (Panax ginseng) – Asian Red Ginseng is an aphrodisiac that increases general energy levels and enhances blood flow to the penis.
- Saw Palmetto (Fructus serenoae) – Often used as a treatment for prostate issues, Saw Palmetto also helps to increase blood flow to the penis, balances hormonal levels, and is used for strengthening and building of body tissues.

- Muira Pauma Bark Extract (Ptychopetalum olacoides) – Restores sexual desire and virility, while increasing the ability to attain and keep an erection.
- Catuaba Bark Extract (Erythroxylum catuaba) – Catuaba is used as an aphrodisiac. It also dilates blood vessels and stimulates the nervous system.
- Hawthorn Berry (Fuctus Crataigi) – Relaxes and dilates arteries, while increasing blood flow.
- Tongkat Ali (Eurycoma longifolia) – This small tree from Southeast Asia provides help as an aphrodisiac and a cure for impotence. It also helps to enhance stamina and strength, increase testosterone, and enhances rigidity, or hardness, in erections.
- Tribulus terrestris is used as an aphrodisiac and testosterone builder and helps to increase pleasure.
- Lepidium meyenii or maca is a plant that is found in Peru. It is high in nutrients that increase energy and libido. It can also work to elevate mood and reduce stress.
- Cayenne – Cayenne enhances and equalizes blood circulation, and also helps to rebuild tissue.
- Taj and Safflower – Both Taj and safflower are vasodilators, which means that they open up blood vessels and encourage increased blood flow, helping to increase the size of an erection and to sustain it for longer.
- Momordica – This herb helps to increase testosterone, stamina and sexual desire.
- Amla and Apigenin - These help maintain the health of your blood vessels.
- Arjuna - Often used in conjunction with amla and apigenin, arjuna regulates heart rate and blood pressure.
- Pygeum Africanum Bark – This bark is used for prostate health.
- Stinging Nettle – Stinging nettle is used for prostate health.

That's a long list! You won't find each of these ingredients in your chosen penis enlargement supplement, but you'll find some of them. The point here is that supplements and their ingredients are used to do several things: increase blood flow, increase tissue health, increase testosterone, increase stamina, build tissue, and increase libido.

These aren't necessarily going to contribute directly to making your penis larger, but they will help make your erections much stronger and add to the possibility of an increase in penile tissue over time. Having more sexual stamina and strength is also a benefit that you may also enjoy from taking a penis enhancement supplement.

Along with what I've listed, you may find additional ingredients such as vitamins and minerals. Often the benefits of penis enlargement pills go beyond making your penis bigger, or your erections more strong and lasting.

Supplements may also help you feel more energetic in general and help to boost your mood. These are good additional benefits from penis supplements, which can help you to feel more confident about yourself and your outlook even before you notice that your penis is getting larger or performing better.

You may also find that your immune system is strengthened resulting in better overall health.

Penis Enlargement Patches

A fairly new development in the penis enhancement field is the use of patches – sort of like the ones you might use to quit smoking.

The whole premise of using a patch to enlarge your penis is that you don't have to take pills, you can put the patch somewhere where no one else will see it and ask about it. The ingredients are delivered transdermal, meaning that they bypass the process of being digested and then moved around your body by your bloodstream.

With patches, the active ingredients (which will be much the same as what you find in pills) are delivered straight into your bloodstream, without delay. Additionally, patches deliver enlarging and enhancing ingredients in a time-released manner, so you get the benefit of them consistently, rather than all at once, as in when you take a pill.

Follow the dosage instructions on the package – some patches last twenty-four hours and some last up to seventy-two hours. And remember these two things: don't put patches in the same place every time and don't put them on a part of your body that is hairy (Ouch!). If you're a pretty hairy guy, you might want to consider shaving an inconspicuous spot or two.

Using Weights and/or a Frame to Stretch Your Penis

Hanging a weight, or weights from you penis to stretch it is a technique (called appropriately enough, hanging) that has been used for a very long time. Enlarging your penis like this can work, but it mostly works for length – if it adds girth, it will be minimal, so keep that in mind if you're thinking of using this method for getting a bigger member.

Now, there is nothing at all wrong with having a long sex organ! But girth is also valued, and that's why most experts don't recommend using weights to stretch out your penis as your only way to make it bigger.

Since we're talking about stretching your penis, one of your most highly regarded body parts, you don't want to do anything that might cause harm, so you need to understand "hanging" before you go and tie a bowling ball to your member. Also, keep in mind that hanging can take weeks or months to work, just like all other penis enlargement programs, so don't get in a hurry with it.

So, how does hanging work anyway? The tissues of your penis, just like any of the soft tissues of your body are very adaptable and will allow themselves to be stretched and manipulated over a period of time.

When you stretch your penis, you'll find that it will become longer and that when you become erect, there is more room to be filled by blood. You may also find that the corpus cavernosum and the corpus spongiosum have increased in area, meaning that the may be some increase in overall bulk.

There are definite risks to hanging. If you use too much weight, you could permanently damage your penis. If the weights are attached incorrectly, blood flow could be reduced to the area, causing terrible consequences.

You can use a similar technique for getting a longer penis without using weights. This is simply stretching your penis by placing it in a frame that has adjustable arms that allow you to gradually lengthen the stretch, and thus, lengthen your penis.

There are kits available that give you everything you need to stretch your penis with or without weights. Generally, a kit will include a frame that you place on your member, weights, and instructions. Kits are also available that you can use for stretching your penis without using weights.

Whether you're hanging with weights, or using only a stretching device, enlarging your penis like this is something that takes hours each day for at least several weeks, and probably several months. Unless you have that kind of time to have a device attached to your organ, hanging and stretching most likely isn't going to be for you.

Using a Pump to Enlarge Your Penis

There has been some question about using pumps to enlarge the penis permanently. We know that pumps can be very effective for men with erectile dysfunction who want to get a good, hard erection. And they can also work for men who have no real problem getting hard, but want to make that erection even harder and bigger. Pumps are great for both purposes.

But can you get lasting results in the bigger organ department with a pump? The answer is yes. Because a pump works the tissues of the penis to expand so they can fill with more blood, eventually, that tissue is going to grow. That's the good news about penis pumps!

The not-so-great news is that if you want to get permanent results from a penis pump, you have to use it every day. It's not going to work like that if you use it just two or three times a week.

Pumps will give you a larger harder erection even if you use them only for when you're actually going to have sex, but when you use a pump only occasionally, the results will be temporary, even if they are impressive.

Penis pumps can also be rather expensive and they have the potential for bursting blood vessels and damaging nerves if not used correctly.

So if you're thinking that a penis pump is the right choice for you, remember that you must, must, must be careful with it so you don't do some major damage to yourself, and that you have to use it almost every day to get the kind of results you want.

Chapter 12: When to Seek Medical Advice

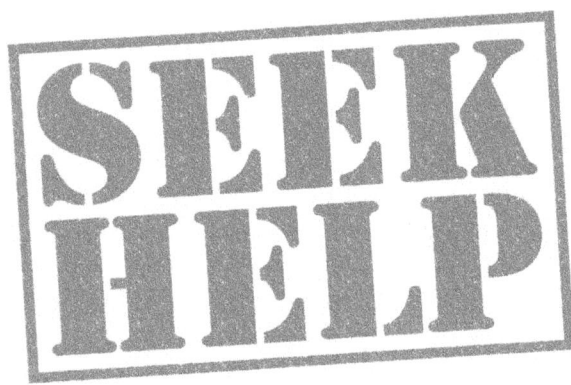

While your penis size is probably within the norm, there are sometimes concerns related to the penis and sexual function that require treatment from a medical professional.

Let's take a look at some issues that require professional help.

Micropenis

There is a true condition where a man's penis is considered less than normal. If your penis measures under three inches when it's erect, you can talk with your physician about possible help.

An urologist can go over options you have to increase the size of your penis slightly so that you can have more successful intercourse. Most likely you'll be offered some surgical options that are really only appropriate if you truly need them.

Erectile Dysfunction

Another problem that can happen for men is erectile dysfunction. This may mean that you're unable to get an erection at all or that you're able to get an erection, but not able to maintain it long enough for intercourse.

Erectile dysfunction is generally a result of poor circulation to the genitals. This can actually be a symptom of a more serious issue such as heart disease. You need to talk to your doctor if you're having trouble with erections.

This problem can also be related to anxiety. If you lack confidence about your size, you may actually have a hard time with erections for psychological reasons.

Treatment for erectile dysfunction can include:

- Therapy to address issues of anxiety
- Medications to improve circulation
- Vacuum pumps to draw blood flow
- Improving your lifestyle for better heart health
- Medications that control blood pressure and cholesterol

Erectile dysfunction is a more serious issue than penis size when it comes to your health and sexual satisfaction. Don't ignore this problem and do talk with your doctor about what you can do.

Premature Ejaculation

Premature ejaculation is another problem related to your penis that's more significant than size. This means that you ejaculate earlier than you would like during sexual intercourse.

For a doctor to diagnose you with premature ejaculation you need to meet the following criteria:

- You almost always ejaculate within a minute of the onset of intercourse
- You're not able to control ejaculation enough to delay it most of the time
- You feel frustrated and stressed about it and therefore avoid sexual activity

If these are common factors for you, your doctor might be able to help you with this situation. This can be caused by physical problems as well as factors related to your psyche.

There are several ways you may be treated for premature ejaculation including:

- Topical creams that cause numbing to slow down stimulation
- Talk therapy to deal with anxiety
- A technique called pause-squeeze that prevents ejaculation
- Antidepressants
- Medications that are used to treat erectile dysfunction in some cases

If you're having problems with premature ejaculation, there's no need to suffer in silence. Unlike penis size, this is a problem that can be easily corrected and you can go onto have a fulfilling sex life for both you and your partner.

Low Libido

You may also notice that you have trouble with your sex drive. This is another issue that is easily corrected with the right help. There are several possible underlying causes for this problem.

You may have psychological issues that are affecting your sex drive such as stress and anxiety – even if it has nothing to do with your sex life. You may also have relationship problems that make it difficult to have sexual intimacy.

Hormones can also be the culprit when it comes to low libido. If your testosterone levels are too low you may not experience as much sexual desire. Your doctor can test your hormone levels and help to correct them if they're not in the normal range.

Some medical conditions such as diabetes, obesity, high cholesterol, and even some medications can also cause problems with your sex drive. By treating the illness or changing your medication you may be able to go right back to your normal desires.

Finally, you may have low levels of dopamine in your brain that keeps you from being able to experience a normal sex drive. For example, patients with Parkinson's disease often have a lower sex drive because of low dopamine levels.

But when medications that stimulate the brain to produce dopamine are introduced, your sex drive may return to normal.

If you feel like your sex drive is suffering, you need to talk with your healthcare provider to rule out serious medical conditions. Together with your doctor you can determine the best course of testing and treatment to help you regain a normal, healthy sex drive.

Male Orgasmic Disorder

It's possible for men to be able to have erections and sexual intercourse, but not achieve an orgasm. There can be psychological as well as physiological causes for this.

Stress and anxiety can cause you to have problems reaching orgasm. So if you're spending a lot of time and energy fretting about your penis size it could eventually lead to this problem.

Sexual trauma such as abuse or rape can also lead to problems with reaching an orgasm. If you've experienced those in your life, speaking with a professional counselor can help you to deal with your feelings and help restore normal sexual function.

You may also have trouble with orgasm if you drink too much alcohol or use other depressive drugs. People who suffer from diabetes and multiple sclerosis also report problems with achieving orgasm.

Finally, you may have experienced an injury or have hormonal problems that keep you from achieving orgasm easily. But for many of these issues there is treatment to help restore sexual function.

Priapsim

Priapism is another condition that is abnormal. In this situation, you actually get a persistent erection that can become painful and last for hours – even with no sexual stimulation.

This can be caused by diseases such as sickle cell anemia. In fact, many men who have sickle cell anemia have this problem. Some medications can also cause you to have this problem.

Illicit drugs such as cocaine and marijuana, black widow spider bites, and carbon monoxide poisoning have also been shown to cause this problem. This is actually a dangerous condition if it's left untreated.

If you experience a painful erection that last more than four hours, you need to seek immediate help – even going to the emergency room. This condition can usually be treated easily and your sexual function will return to normal – and most important you can get relief from the pain and swelling.

CHAPTER 13: DIET, EXERCISE AND YOUR HEALTH

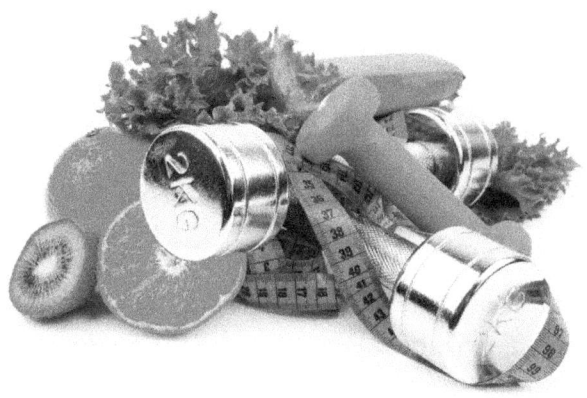

If you're wondering why there's a chapter about your health in this book, think of it this way: a person can have three million in the bank, and not be healthy at all. That person isn't really going to enjoy all that money if he or she is sick, nor is that person going to be able to make more money to add to the three million.

Or how about this: a woman has a really pretty face and gorgeous hair, but she's not looking good at all in the body department – she's waaaay too skinny or waaaay overweight. It's not an optimal situation.

One more example: You grow your penis to a great size, and your erections are stupendous. But you're out of shape – just going up a flight of stairs tires you out. Hmmmm.

See where we're headed? You need the whole package to be healthy and in shape for you to fully enjoy the benefits of developing that nice big penis.

Do you have to be Mr. Universe? No! Do you have to turn into a vegetarian, health-food nut? No!

You just have to remember that your food choices, good nutrition, healthy habits and a whole body exercise plan is going to help you:

1. Get the penis you want
2. Enjoy the penis you get

So, we're going to discuss your diet, fitness and health before this book comes to an end.

Habits That Negatively Effect Your Penis, Your Sex Life and Your Health

I'm not going to pull any punches here, but am just going to tell it like it is. There are habits in your lifestyle that are not good for your general health and that are disasters for your penis.

You might not realize it right now, but I guarantee you that if you make healthy changes in your lifestyle, you will feel better all over, and you'll also have better erections, sexual stamina and you'll have much better prospects for growing your penis to a larger size. Here's a list of the habits that you need to change – starting now.

- Smoking – If you don't smoke, congratulations! And for goodness' sake, don't start! If you are a smoker, even only a couple a day, you need to stop! I know that this is much easier said than done, but here's the bad stuff that smoking does to you: ruins your lungs, greatly increases your risk of heart disease and stroke, greatly increases your risk for cancer, makes it harder to breath, can lead to COPD and emphysema, makes you smell bad, can lead to erectile dysfunction.

Whoa! See your doctor to find out about the best way for you to quit smoking. If you try to quit and aren't successful, try again. And keep trying!

- Alcohol Abuse – A drink now and then is fine – as long as you're not using drinking to self-medicate or for the sole purpose of getting drunk. Drinking and driving is never okay.

Acting like an idiot because you're drunk makes you lose friends and the respect of others. And abusing alcohol can lead to higher risk of certain types of cancer, liver disease, brain damage, and suppressed immune system and legal problems. On top of that, can help cause erectile dysfunction!

If you have trouble knowing when to stop drinking, get help. See your doctor or other health professional.

- Lack of Exercise – Regular exercise is the cornerstone of a healthy life. We're not talking only about exercising your penis and your PC muscle. This is about getting regular exercise that raises your heart rate and gets your whole body working.

Regular exercise will help you regulate and/or lose weight and keep your immune system in tune. It will also help protect you against heart disease, and all sorts of illnesses and injuries.

Getting consistent exercise will also slow your body's aging process. It regulates circulation and gives you more energy and stamina. If you need to lose some weight because your belly fat is making your penis looks smallish, exercise is an important part of that process.

- Poor Nutrition – Ever since you were a wee little boy, your mom, dad, grandmother and probably every other adult you knew tried to get you to eat your broccoli. They were right. A proper diet, with a good variety of food and balance of nutrients will boost your health, help you lose and regulate your weight and give you more energy.

Concentrate your eating habits on lean proteins, less red meat, more fruits and vegetables, low-fat dairy, lots of water, and complex carbohydrates. Stay away from processed sugar, too much salt, too much caffeine, candy and sweet, and trans-fats and hydrogenated fats. Leave the junk food and fast food alone!

- Stress – Stress can cause erectile dysfunction. It can also contribute to a weakened immune system, heart disease and stroke, cancer and other illnesses. Stress happens to everyone, and more and more, we lead stressful lives.

It's important to keep your lifestyle and eating habits as healthy as possible to help reverse the effects of stress. You can also practice stress relieving techniques such as doing yoga or Tai chi, deep breathing or even seeing a counselor on a regular basis to just unload your concerns about life and learn new ways of absorbing and combating stress and stressful situations.

- Lack of Sleep – Your body needs a minimum of six hours of sleep per night. A minimum. Some people need eight to nine hours of sleep every night. If you regularly don't get enough sleep, you're setting yourself up for illness.

You're also setting yourself up for failure at your penis enlargement program because you'll be too tired to be consistent with it, and your body won't be able to respond as well to the exercises because it will be trying to conserve it's energy because you're not sleeping enough. Get your rest!

A Proper Diet for Health and Fitness

Let's look a bit more closely at what a proper diet for health and fitness would look like. You need to pay close attention to your diet, especially now for a couple reasons.

First, your penis is going to automatically look larger when your abdominal area is trimmer. Simple as that. Second, good nutrition is the basis for building muscle, tissue and strength – all things that you're trying to do with your enlargement program, right?

Without a healthy plan for proper eating, you might not be giving your body what it really needs to help make that sex organ bigger.

Vitamin and mineral supplements can help, but your best source for good nutrition is healthy food.

So, let's take a bit of time to look at what you should eat and what you shouldn't eat.

Proteins

Proteins help in cell and tissue growth. They are building blocks for your body, so you can already see why they are going to be important to you in your penis enhancement program.

You might think of protein being supplied mainly by meats, but you can also find protein in other sources, such as soy products, eggs, nuts, dairy products and beans. Protein drinks and bars are ready made ways to get a quick and convenient serving of protein.

As a general rule, a healthy adult needs about eight grams of protein per pound of body weight, per day. If you're exercising vigorously (as in going to the gym every day and working out, or jogging every day, or similar), you'll need closer to one and a half grams per day.

You shouldn't overdo it on protein, though. While it's vital to your health, too much is very hard on your liver and kidneys, organs that bear the brunt of processing the by-products of protein rich foods.

Fruits and Vegetables

These are essential for providing vitamins and minerals, not to mention fiber to your diet. Most people forget to eat enough fruits and vegetables - you should have at least three fruit servings and five vegetable servings a day.

Besides providing vitamins and minerals in large quantities, they provide energy and help you feel full – this is really important if you're trying to shed a few pounds.

Complex Carbohydrates

You need carbohydrates because they provide energy. Simple carbs, like white bread provide energy in one big shot and then leave you feeling lethargic. Additionally, they are overly processed and have little nutritional value.

Complex carbs, like whole grain breads, rolls, pastas and cereals are excellent for providing sustained energy and fiber that helps to fill you up and keep your digestive system working well.

Low-Fat Dairy

Dairy is good for you, unless you're allergic to milk products. They provide calcium and vitamin D for strong bones. They also provide protein. Regular dairy is high in fat. Choose low-fat dairy products to keep from gaining unnecessary weight and clogging your arteries. Generally speaking, the only people who need regular dairy, with all the fat, are children.

If you're allergic to milk, try soy dairy products.

Fats

Small amounts of healthy fats are necessary in everyone's diet. Fats help with cell metabolism, the manufacture and regulation of hormones, and regulating blood clogging.

Choose healthy fats, in small amounts. This includes virgin olive oil, flax oil, safflower oil, hemp seed oil, walnut and wheat germ oil. You can also eat fish such as salmon, mackerel, tuna and sardines to get healthy servings of omega-3 oils in your diet.

Drink Lots of Water

Keep your body hydrated with plenty of fresh, pure water. Water helps your body function at optimal health and performance. A general rule is eight – eight ounces glasses a day. You'll need more if you exercise vigorously or live in a hot climate. Stay hydrated!

Foods to Avoid

There has already been some mention of this earlier, but it bears repeating. Foods that are full of sugar, simple carbohydrates, highly processed foods, soda, caffeine, alcohol, fatty foods, foods from fast food restaurants, and lots of salt (substitute with sea salt when possible, but still limit it), should all be eaten in limited quantities or not at all. These foods won't do anything to help your health or your penis growth.

If you haven't been eating a balanced, healthy diet, you might find these changes difficult at first. Rest assured that as you stick with a healthy eating plan, your body will respond in a positive manner by losing excess weight, having more energy and just plain feeling better. You'll also notice that cravings for sugar and salt diminish.

General Fitness

What good is a super-sized penis going to be if the rest of your is out of shape?

General fitness should be every adults concern. A reasonable level of fitness brings many benefits. First off, you'll look better. The more fit you are, the better your clothes will look on you, and the better you'll look without them on!

Good fitness also translates into confidence. It's no secret that men who are physically fit are more confident not only in the bedroom, but the boardroom, the garage, and a Saturday night out on the town. Physical fitness helps you feel better about yourself in a multitude of ways – it psychologically creates a better outlook that you can benefit from.

Did you know that regular exercise boosts your mood and helps protect you from many types of disease? Did you know that it can help you look younger as you age? Did you know that regular exercise helps you get a better night's sleep? It does all that and more!

I'm not going to tell you how to exercise, or when to exercise. All I'm going to recommend here is that you do exercise a minimum of 30 minutes a day, at least three days a week. Your activity level should be at least moderate, meaning that it should make your heart rate increase as well as your breathing, and you should feel like you've done something when you're finished.

The good news is that you don't have to get that whole thirty minutes done at one time. Three sessions of ten minutes will work, too.

Note: thirty minutes is the minimum. It's better to get forty-five 45 to sixty minutes of exercise per day, three to five days a week.

Now I realize that you're already doing your penis enlargement exercises and that they take time. But full body exercise is also an investment in your future health and happiness, so it's vital.

If you're not used to getting regular exercise, it may take some time for you to find the right fit. Try a variety of forms of exercise out. If you don't feel you can afford a gym membership, you can swim (if there is a pool available) walk, bike or jog your way to fitness. Walking your dog at a swift pace every day will do wonders!

Sports that keep you moving are great, so hit the basketball or tennis court!

If you decided to join a gym, do a variety of exercises and include both aerobic exercise and weights in your routine. You might want to have a trainer help you for a couple sessions, so you know the correct techniques.

Regardless of how you do it, get off the sofa and away from your TV and computer and MOVE!

Chapter 14: Conclusion

Above and beyond all else, it's vital that you know that you can have a larger penis. There are many ways to accomplish this goal. Yes, they all take time, but that's just the way it is.

If you're looking for a miracle, as in several more inches in a week, you're going to be sorely disappointed. If you're realistic and do the work, you'll be pleased to see that over a period of weeks and months, your penis will be both longer and thicker forever.

This book has provided you with the information you need to get started. Now it's up to you to do the work. Stay motivated.

Take good care of your body through proper diet and exercise and stick with your enlargement program and you'll see results.

Don't forget that there are a multitude of things you can do to and with your partner, or future partner, in bed. While your member is important, it's not the only thing you have to work with. Take time to learn sexual techniques that will keep her satisfied. Your hands and mouth, your imagination and your words all work together to bring pleasure, too.

And remember this, also. With many women, sex begins way before you get to the bedroom. It begins with a sly glance across a table, or your hand resting gently on the small of her back. Your sense of humor or kindness towards others might be part of what turns her on and makes her want to get naked with you.

While your penis is very, very important, it's not the only thing she thinks about when it comes to sex.

As you enlarge your penis, take time to study sex techniques and give some thought to the art of seduction. By the time you've gained the inches you want, you'll be prepared to greet the world as the sex god that you are!

Good luck in your enhancement endeavors and all your life goals. Confidence and a can-do attitude is your first step!

www.ingramcontent.com/pod-product-compliance
Ingram Content Group UK Ltd.
Pitfield, Milton Keynes, MK11 3LW, UK
UKHW022221230426
12048UKWH00016BA/986